VALVULAR HEART DISEASE

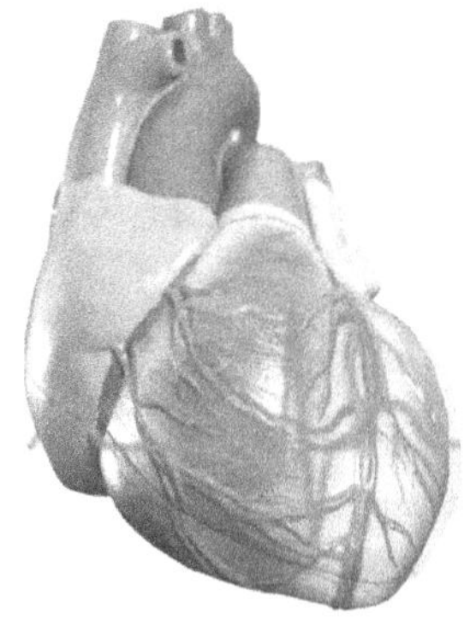

A Simple Guide To Understanding And Managing Valvular Heart Disease

By

Dr. Givens Bestman

DISCLAIMER

Copyright © Dr. Givens Bestman 2024. All Rights Reserved.

No part of this publication may be reproduced, distributed, or transmitted in any form or by any means, including photocopying, recording, or other electronic or mechanical methods, without the prior written permission of the publisher, except in the case of brief quotations embodied in critical reviews and certain other noncommercial uses permitted by copyright law.

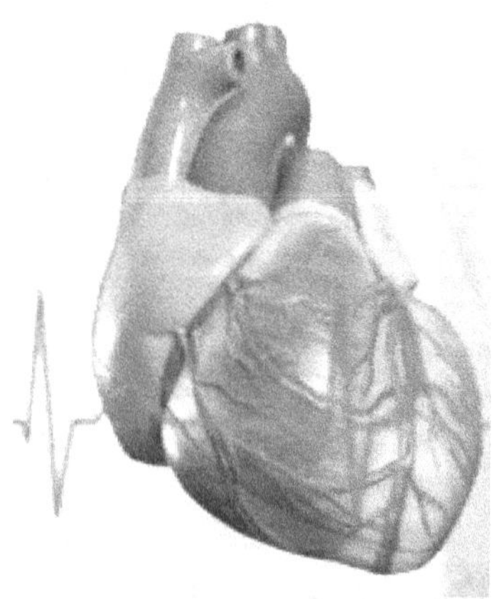

Table of Contents

INTRODUCTION

Samantha is the only daughter in a family of six, loved dearly by her parents and siblings. This family of six lived a quiet life in a small town. Samantha, got married to Mr. Ben, and moved to another town where her heartthrob, Mr. Ben secured a good job to carter for them.

After six years of marriage with two beautiful daughters, Samantha was diagnosed with valvular heart disease. She chose to keep this burden to herself, shielding her family, especially her aged parents, from the worry and fear that such news might instill, bravely battling the illness for eight long months.

Samantha's husband, Mr. Ben, noticed the toll the condition was taking on his beloved wife. Driven by concern and love, he embarked on an exhaustive journey of research, delving into articles and consulting with health practitioners to find a way to restore Samantha's health and bring happiness back to their family.

After months of research, near despair and was on the verge of breaking his promise to Samantha. The burden of the secret and the fear of losing his wife were almost too much to bear. Mr. Ben stumbled upon a beacon of hope — "Valvular Heart Disease: A Simple Guide to Understanding and Managing Valvular Heart Disease." As he devoured its pages with enthusiasm, a newfound sense of hope and understanding washed over him. Armed with knowledge, he rushed home to Samantha, delivering the news that would change their lives.

Samantha, with the guidance from the valuable insights in the guide, started to recover. The couple, now armed with a plan and newfound hope, decided to break the news to Samantha's family during their yearly get-together. To their astonishment, they discovered that Samantha's elder brother, Martins, was also suffering from the same condition, he was diagnosed barely a month to the get-together

The family, now equipped with knowledge from the guide, faced the challenge head-on. Samantha and Martins, supported by Mr. Ben and their family, underwent the necessary treatments and lifestyle adjustments outlined in the guide. The guide became their trusted companion, providing clarity and direction in their battle against valvular heart disease.

In the end, the family emerged victorious. Samantha and Martins not only conquered their health struggles but also became advocates for awareness and understanding of valvular heart disease. The simple guide that once saved Samantha's life became a beacon of hope for their entire family, underscoring the importance of knowledge, support, and resilience in the face of adversity.

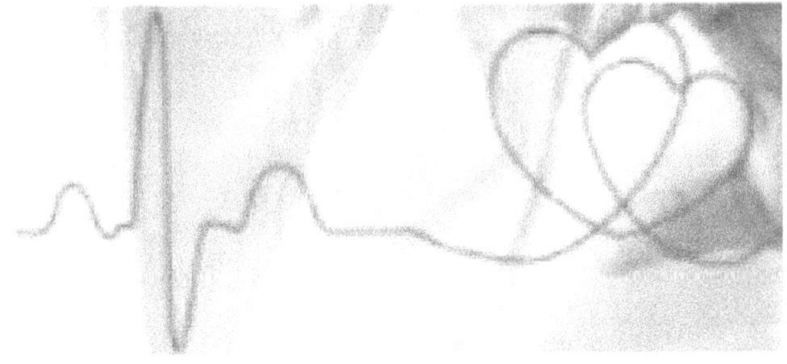

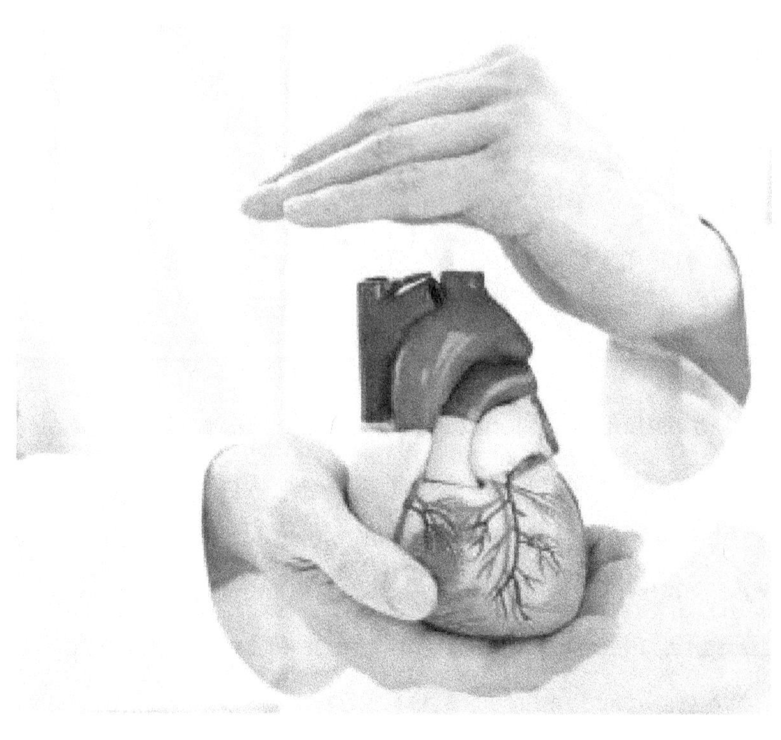

CHAPTER 1

Definition of Valvular Heart Disease

Valvular heart disease is a medical condition characterized by abnormalities in the heart valves, which are responsible for regulating the flow of blood within the heart. The heart valves ensure that blood moves through the heart in one direction, preventing any backward flow. When these valves become damaged, narrowed (stenosis), or fail to close properly (regurgitation), it disrupts the normal blood flow.

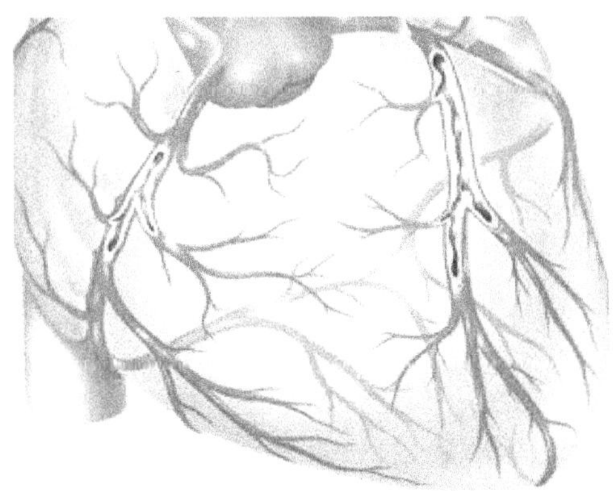

Anatomy and Function of Heart Valves

The heart is a sophisticated organ that pumps blood to the lungs and the body, where it is deoxygenated. The proper functioning of the heart valves is crucial for maintaining the unidirectional flow of blood through the four chambers of the heart. Here is an overview of the anatomy and function of the heart valves:

1. Mitral Valve: The mitral valve, also known as the bicuspid valve, is located between the left atrium and the left ventricle. It consists of two leaflets, or flaps, which open and close to allow blood to flow from the left atrium into the left ventricle during diastole (relaxation phase) and prevent backflow during systole (contraction phase). The mitral valve plays a key role in regulating the flow of oxygenated blood from the lungs into the systemic circulation.

2. Tricuspid Valve: The tricuspid valve is situated between the right atrium and the right ventricle. It is composed of three leaflets and functions similarly to the mitral valve.

During diastole, the tricuspid valve opens to allow blood to flow from the right atrium into the right ventricle, while during systole, it closes to prevent the backward flow of blood.

3. Aortic Valve: The aortic valve is located between the left ventricle and the aorta, the main artery that carries oxygenated blood to the body. It consists of three leaflets and opens during systole to allow blood to be ejected from the left ventricle into the aorta. When the ventricle relaxes during diastole, the aortic valve closes, preventing blood from flowing back into the ventricle.

4. Pulmonary Valve: The right ventricle and the pulmonary artery, which carries deoxygenated blood to the lungs for oxygenation, are separated by the pulmonary valve. Similar to the aortic valve, it has three leaflets and opens during systole to allow blood to be pumped from the right ventricle into the pulmonary artery. During diastole, the pulmonary valve closes, preventing the backflow of blood into the ventricle.

Structure of Heart Valves

Heart valves are intricate structures composed of specialized tissues designed to facilitate the unidirectional flow of blood through the heart. Each valve consists of several components that work together to ensure efficient and coordinated functioning. Here is a brief overview of the structure of heart valves:

1. Leaflets/Flaps: The leaflets, also known as flaps, are the primary components of heart valves. They are thin, flexible structures that open and close to regulate blood flow. The number of leaflets varies depending on the valve. For instance, the mitral and tricuspid valves have two and three leaflets, respectively, while the aortic and pulmonary valves have three leaflets each.

2. Annulus: The annulus is the fibrous ring-like structure that surrounds the valve opening. It provides stability and serves as an attachment point for the valve leaflets.
The annulus ensures proper positioning and function of the valve.

3. Chordae Tendineae: Chordae tendineae are strong, fibrous cords that connect the valve leaflets to the papillary muscles within the ventricles. These tendons prevent the leaflets from prolapsing (bulging backward) into the atria during ventricular contraction. They maintain proper alignment and tension, allowing the valve to open and close effectively.

4. Papillary Muscles: Papillary muscles are specialized muscles located within the ventricles of the heart. They attach to the chordae tendineae and contract during ventricular systole (contraction phase). The contraction of papillary muscles pulls on the chordae tendineae, exerting tension on the valve leaflets and preventing them from reversing into the atria.

5. Valve Endothelium: The valve endothelium is a thin layer of specialized endothelial cells that line the inner surface of the valve leaflets.

These cells provide a smooth surface that minimizes friction and promotes efficient blood flow. They also play a role in maintaining the integrity and function of the valve.

6. Supporting Connective Tissue: Heart valves contain connective tissue that provides structural support and elasticity. The connective tissue helps maintain the shape and integrity of the valve leaflets, allowing them to withstand the pressure changes that occur during each cardiac cycle.

Damage or abnormalities in any of these components can affect the proper functioning of the valves, leading to conditions such as stenosis (narrowing) or regurgitation (leaking).

Importance of Heart Valve Health

Maintaining healthy heart valves is crucial for the proper functioning of the cardiovascular system. The valves play a vital role in ensuring unidirectional blood flow through the heart chambers, optimizing cardiac output, and preventing backflow or regurgitation. Here is an overview of the importance of heart valve health:

1. Uninterrupted Blood Flow: Heart valves ensure the smooth and uninterrupted flow of blood through the heart. Properly functioning valves allow blood to move efficiently from one chamber to another without obstruction or leakage. This unidirectional flow ensures that oxygenated blood is effectively delivered to the body's organs and tissues while deoxygenated blood is directed to the lungs for oxygenation.

2. Optimal Cardiac Output: Heart valves contribute to maintaining optimal cardiac output, which is the volume of blood pumped by the heart per minute. By opening and closing at precise times during the cardiac cycle, the valves allow the heart to efficiently pump blood.
Any dysfunction or obstruction in the valves can reduce cardiac output, leading to symptoms such as fatigue, shortness of breath, and decreased exercise tolerance.

3. Prevention of Backflow and Regurgitation: The valves prevent the backflow or regurgitation of blood. They close tightly during ventricular contraction, preventing blood from flowing back into the atria.

This ensures that blood is propelled forward into the systemic and pulmonary circulations. Regurgitation, caused by valve dysfunction, can lead to volume overload, increased workload on the heart, and compromised cardiac function.

4. Maintenance of Hemodynamic Balance: Healthy heart valves contribute to maintaining hemodynamic balance within the heart.

They assist in maintaining appropriate pressures within the chambers, preventing excessive pressure build-up or backflow that can strain the heart and compromise its function. Proper valve function helps maintain efficient blood circulation and minimizes stress on the heart muscle.

5. Prevention of Complications: Maintaining healthy heart valves helps prevent potential complications associated with valvular heart diseases. Valve abnormalities, such as stenosis or regurgitation, can lead to symptoms, such as heart failure, arrhythmias, blood clots, and infective endocarditis.

Timely detection and appropriate management of valve conditions can help reduce the risk of complications and improve overall prognosis.

6. Quality of Life: Heart valve health directly impacts an individual's quality of life. Proper valve function allows for normal physical activity, adequate oxygenation of tissues, and overall well-being. Valve diseases, if left untreated, can significantly impair daily activities, limit exercise capacity, and reduce overall quality of life.

Regular medical check-ups, prompt diagnosis, and appropriate management of heart valve conditions are essential for maintaining valve health and preventing complications.

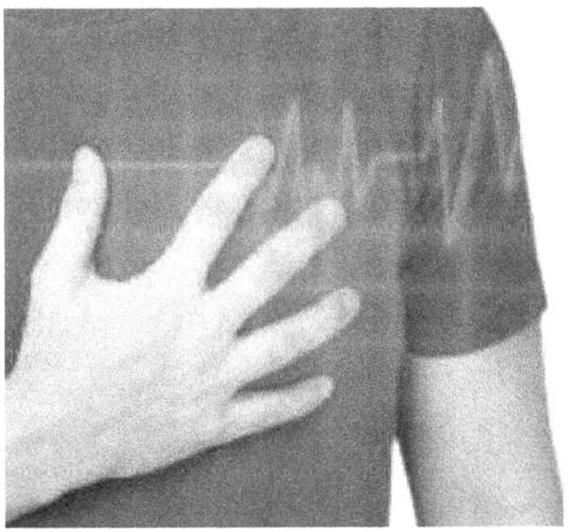

Lifestyle modifications, Medication management, and, in some cases, Surgical interventions can help preserve or restore proper valve function, ensuring optimal cardiovascular health and well-being.

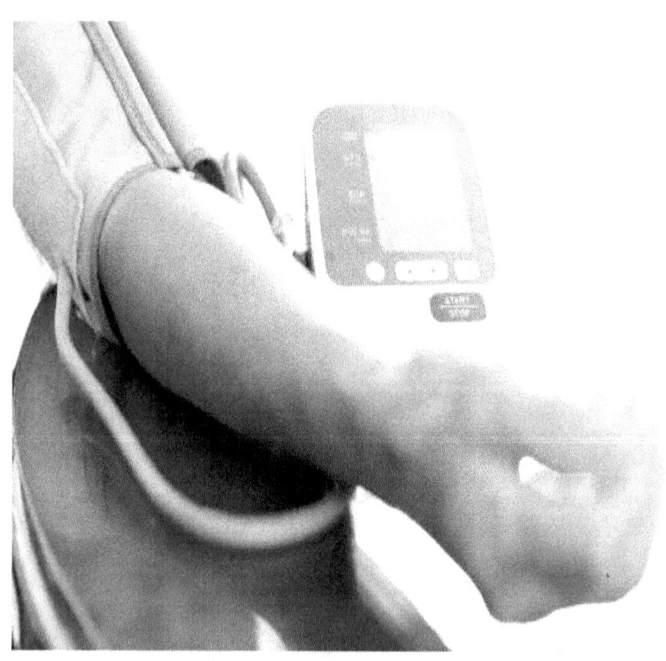

CHAPTER 2

Common Valvular Heart Diseases

Valvular heart diseases encompass a range of conditions that affect the normal functioning of the heart valves. These conditions can lead to impaired blood flow, resulting in symptoms and potential complications. Overview of some common valvular heart diseases:

1. Mitral Valve Stenosis: Mitral valve stenosis occurs when the mitral valve, situated between the left atrium and left ventricle, becomes narrowed. This narrowing restricts blood flow from the left atrium to the left ventricle, leading to increased pressure in the left atrium and potential congestion in the lungs. Mitral valve stenosis is commonly caused by rheumatic fever, a complication of untreated streptococcal throat infection.

2. Mitral Valve Regurgitation: Mitral valve regurgitation, also known as mitral insufficiency or mitral incompetence, is characterized by the incomplete closure of the mitral valve.

This results in the backward flow of blood from the left ventricle to the left atrium during systole. Mitral valve regurgitation can be caused by mitral valve prolapse, rheumatic heart disease, infective endocarditis, or other structural abnormalities.

3. Aortic Valve Stenosis: Aortic valve stenosis occurs when the aortic valve, situated between the left ventricle and the aorta, becomes narrowed, obstructing the blood flow from the left ventricle to the aorta. Aortic valve stenosis is commonly caused by age-related degeneration, calcification of the valve leaflets, or congenital abnormalities. It can lead to left ventricular hypertrophy and reduced cardiac output.

4. Aortic Valve Regurgitation: Aortic valve regurgitation, also known as aortic insufficiency, is characterized by the inability of the aortic valve to close properly. This allows blood to leak back into the left ventricle during diastole. Aortic valve regurgitation can be caused by various factors, including aortic root dilation, infective endocarditis, rheumatic heart disease, or congenital abnormalities.

5. Tricuspid Valve Regurgitation: Tricuspid valve regurgitation occurs when the tricuspid valve, located between the right atrium and right ventricle, fails to close tightly. This results in the backward flow of blood from the right ventricle to the right atrium during systole. Tricuspid valve regurgitation can be caused by conditions such as tricuspid valve prolapse, infective endocarditis, or right ventricular dilation.

6. Pulmonary Valve Stenosis: Pulmonary valve stenosis involves the narrowing of the pulmonary valve, situated between the right ventricle and the pulmonary artery. This narrowing restricts the blood flow from the right ventricle to the lungs, leading to increased pressure in the right ventricle. Pulmonary valve stenosis can be caused by congenital malformations or acquired conditions. These common valvular heart diseases can range in severity from mild to severe.

Chapter 3

Signs and Symptoms of Valvular Heart Disease

Valvular heart disease refers to conditions that affect the heart valves, impairing their normal function and disrupting blood flow through the heart. The signs and symptoms can vary depending on the specific valve affected and the severity of the disease. Here is a short and detailed overview of the signs and symptoms commonly associated with valvular heart disease:

1. Heart Murmur: One of the hallmark signs of valvular heart disease is the presence of a heart murmur. A heart murmur is an abnormal sound heard during a physical examination when a healthcare provider listens to the heart using a stethoscope. The murmur is caused by turbulent blood flow across a narrowed or leaky valve and can vary in intensity and characteristics depending on the specific valve affected.

2. Chest Pain or Discomfort: Individuals with valvular heart disease may experience chest pain or discomfort. This can occur due to reduced blood flow to the heart muscle or the increased workload on the heart. The pain may be described as a pressure, squeezing, or tightness in the chest and can sometimes radiate to the neck, jaw, arms, or back.

3. Shortness of Breath: Breathlessness or shortness of breath is a common symptom of valvular heart disease. It may occur during physical activity or even at rest, depending on the severity of the valve disease. The reduced cardiac output or increased pressure within the heart chambers can lead to fluid buildup in the lungs, causing difficulty in breathing.

4. Fatigue and Weakness: Valvular heart disease can cause fatigue and weakness. The heart's reduced ability to pump blood efficiently can result in inadequate oxygen and nutrient delivery to the body's organs and tissues, leading to a sense of tiredness and lack of energy.

5. Palpitations and Irregular Heartbeat: Some individuals with valvular heart disease may experience palpitations, which are sensations of a rapid or irregular heartbeat. This can occur due to abnormal electrical conduction in the heart or the compensatory mechanisms the heart employs to maintain adequate blood flow despite the valve dysfunction.

6. Edema and Fluid Retention: Valvular heart disease can lead to fluid retention and swelling in different parts of the body. This is often noticeable in the ankles, feet, legs, or abdomen. The impaired blood flow and increased pressure within the heart chambers can cause fluid to accumulate in the tissues, resulting in edema.

7. Dizziness and Fainting: In severe cases of valvular heart disease, individuals may experience dizziness or fainting episodes. This can occur due to reduced blood flow to the brain, resulting in inadequate oxygen supply. Fainting, also known as syncope, can be a result of arrhythmias or decreased cardiac output.

CHAPTER 4

Diagnosis Of Valvular Heart Disease

The diagnosis of valvular heart disease involves a comprehensive evaluation by healthcare professionals to assess the function and structure of the heart valves. It typically includes a combination of medical history assessment, physical examination, and various diagnostic tests. Here is a short overview of the diagnostic process for valvular heart disease:

1. Medical History: The healthcare provider will take a detailed medical history, including information about symptoms, risk factors, and any previous heart conditions. They will inquire about symptoms such as chest pain, shortness of breath, fatigue, or swelling, as well as any history of infections, rheumatic fever, or other relevant conditions.

2. Physical Examination: During a physical examination, the healthcare provider will listen to the heart using a stethoscope to detect abnormal heart sounds, such as murmurs or other characteristic sounds associated with valvular heart disease. They will also assess other signs such as abnormal heart rhythms, fluid retention (swelling in the extremities or abdomen), or signs of heart failure.

3. Diagnostic Tests:

i. **Echocardiography:** Echocardiography is a key diagnostic test for valvular heart disease. It uses ultrasound waves to create detailed images of the heart and valves. This test can assess valve structure, function, and measure the severity of valve abnormalities.

ii. **Doppler Ultrasound:** Doppler ultrasound is often performed alongside echocardiography to assess blood flow across the heart valves. It provides information about the direction, velocity, and turbulence of blood flow, aiding in the evaluation of valve regurgitation or stenosis.

iii.   **Electrocardiogram (ECG):** An ECG records the electrical activity of the heart and can help identify irregular heart rhythms or signs of strain on the heart muscle caused by valvular heart disease.

iv.   **Chest X-ray:** A chest X-ray may be performed to assess the size and shape of the heart and lungs, which can provide additional information about valve disease and its impact on the heart and lungs.

v.   **Cardiac MRI or CT scan:** In some cases, cardiac magnetic resonance imaging (MRI) or computed tomography (CT) scans may be conducted to obtain more detailed images of the heart valves and surrounding structures.

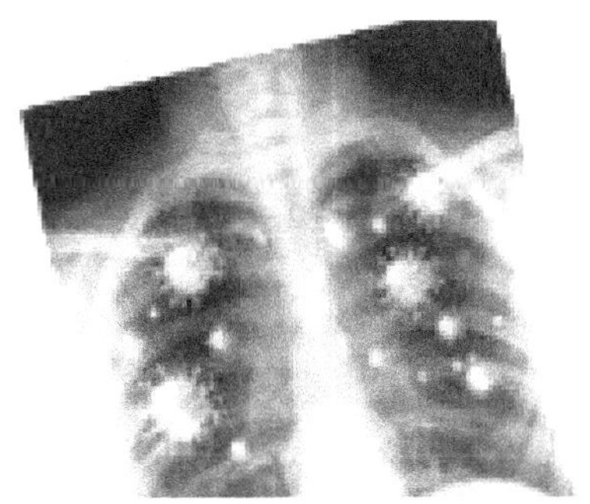

4. Additional Tests: In certain situations, additional tests may be necessary, such as stress tests to evaluate the heart's response to exercise, cardiac catheterization to measure pressures within the heart chambers, or blood tests to assess overall heart function and check for specific markers of valve disease.

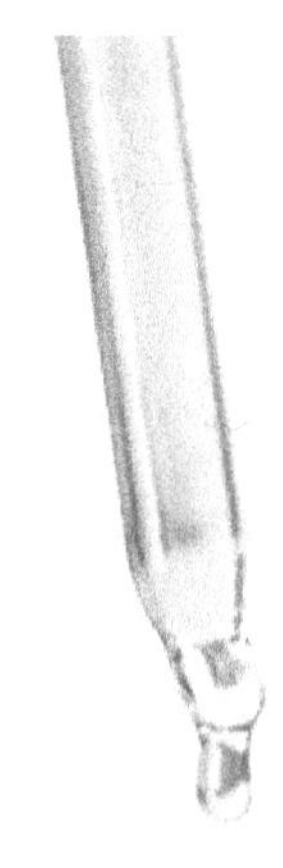

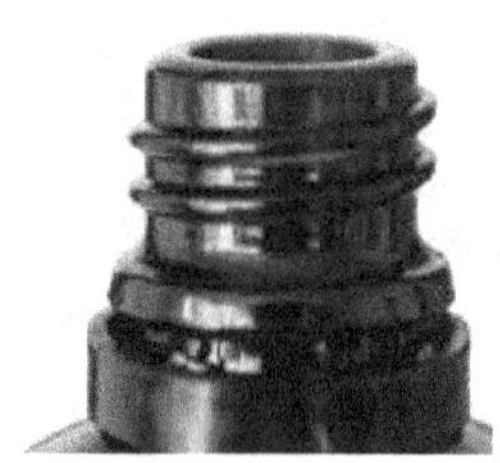

CHAPTER 5

Treatment Options for Valvular Heart Disease

The treatment of valvular heart disease aims to alleviate symptoms, improve quality of life, and prevent or manage complications. The appropriate treatment option depends on factors such as the type and severity of the valve disease, the presence of symptoms, the overall health of the individual, and the risk-benefit assessment by the healthcare team. Here is a short and detailed overview of the treatment options for valvular heart disease:

Medications for Valvular Heart Disease

Medications play an important role in the management of valvular heart disease. They are prescribed to alleviate symptoms, control underlying conditions, prevent complications, and improve overall heart function.

The specific medications prescribed will depend on the type and severity of the valve disease, associated conditions, and individual factors:

1. Diuretics:

- ❖ Diuretics, such as furosemide or hydrochlorothiazide, are commonly prescribed to manage fluid retention and reduce swelling (edema) in valvular heart disease.

   They increase urine production, helping to eliminate excess fluid from the body and relieve symptoms such as shortness of breath and swelling in the legs.

2. Beta-Blockers:

- ❖ Beta-blockers, such as metoprolol or carvedilol, are medications that block the effects of adrenaline on the heart. They help regulate heart rate, reduce blood pressure, and improve the heart's efficiency. Beta-blockers can alleviate symptoms, such as chest pain and palpitations, and are often prescribed to manage valvular heart disease, especially when there is associated hypertension or heart failure.

3. Calcium Channel Blockers:

- ❖ Calcium channel blockers, such as amlodipine or diltiazem, relax and widen blood vessels, reducing the workload on the heart. They can be beneficial in managing symptoms of valvular heart disease, such as chest pain and high blood pressure. Calcium channel blockers are also used for treating certain arrhythmias associated with valvular heart disease.

4. Anticoagulants:

- ❖ Anticoagulant medications, such as warfarin or direct oral anticoagulants (DOACs) like apixaban or rivaroxaban, are prescribed to prevent blood clot formation in individuals with valvular heart disease who are at risk of thromboembolic events. Anticoagulants are particularly important for individuals with mechanical heart valves or atrial fibrillation, as these conditions increase the risk of blood clots.

5. Antiarrhythmics:

❖ Antiarrhythmic medications, such as amiodarone or flecainide, may be prescribed to manage abnormal heart rhythms (arrhythmias) associated with valvular heart disease. These medications help regulate the heart's electrical activity, restoring normal rhythm and reducing symptoms such as palpitations or irregular heartbeat.

6. Medications for Associated Conditions:

❖ Additional medications may be prescribed to manage associated conditions, such as hypertension, heart failure, or coronary artery disease.

These may include ACE inhibitors, angiotensin receptor blockers (ARBs), statins, or medications to optimize blood pressure and overall heart function.

Valve Repair

Valve repair is a surgical procedure commonly performed to treat valvular heart disease. It aims to restore the normal structure and function of a diseased or damaged heart valve, preserving the native valve rather than replacing it with an artificial prosthesis. Here is a detailed overview of valve repair for valvular heart disease:

1. Purpose:

❖ Valve repair is performed to correct abnormalities in the heart valves, such as stenosis (narrowing) or regurgitation (leakage).

The procedure aims to improve valve function, enhance blood flow through the heart, alleviate symptoms, and prevent complications.

2. Surgical Techniques:

The specific technique used for valve repair depends on the type and location of the valve disease. The surgeon may employ various approaches, including:

❖ **Valve Resection:** Removal of diseased or damaged portions of the valve.

- ❖ **Valve Annuloplasty:** Repairing the valve's annulus (the ring-shaped structure supporting the valve) by inserting a flexible or rigid ring to reshape and reinforce it.
- ❖ **Leaflet Repair:** Repairing or reconstructing the valve leaflets to improve their function and ensure proper sealing.

3. Benefits:

Valve repair offers several advantages over valve replacement. These include:

- ❖ **Preserving The Native Valve:** Repairing the existing valve allows for the preservation of the patient's own tissue and avoids the need for lifelong anticoagulation therapy in most cases.
- ❖ **Maintaining Normal Valve Function:** Valve repair aims to restore the valve's normal function, facilitating improved blood flow and preventing the backward flow of blood (regurgitation).

❖ **Long-Term Durability:** Valve repair can provide excellent long-term outcomes and durability, especially in certain valve conditions, such as mitral valve repair for mitral regurgitation.

4. Patient Selection:

Not all valve diseases are suitable for repair, and the decision for valve repair or replacement depends on various factors. These factors include the specific valve involved, the severity and type of valve disease, the patient's overall health, and the experience and expertise of the surgical team. In some cases, valve replacement may be more appropriate.

5. Postoperative Care:

After valve repair surgery, patients will require careful monitoring and follow-up care. This includes regular visits to the healthcare provider, adherence to prescribed medications, and lifestyle modifications to promote heart health. Rehabilitation and cardiac rehabilitation programs may be recommended to aid in recovery and optimize long-term outcomes.

Valve repair is an effective treatment option for select cases of valvular heart disease. It aims to restore the normal function of the valve, improve blood flow, and alleviate symptoms. The decision for valve repair versus replacement is based on individual patient factors and should be discussed with a healthcare provider specializing in valvular heart disease.

Valve Replacement

Valve replacement is a surgical procedure performed to treat valvular heart disease when the damaged valve cannot be repaired.

It involves removing the diseased or malfunctioning valve and replacing it with an artificial prosthesis. Here is a short overview of valve replacement:

1. Purpose:

- Valve replacement is performed to address severe valve abnormalities that cannot be effectively repaired. It aims to restore proper blood flow, alleviate symptoms, and prevent complications associated with valvular heart disease.

2. Types of Valve Prostheses:

There are two main types of valve prostheses used for replacement:

- ❖ **Mechanical Valves**: These valves are made of durable materials, such as carbon or metal alloys, and are designed to last a long time. However, individuals with mechanical valves require lifelong anticoagulation therapy to prevent blood clots.

- ❖ **Biological Valves:** Also known as tissue or bioprosthetic valves, these are typically made from animal tissue (e.g., pig or cow) or, in some cases, human tissue. Biological valves may not require long-term anticoagulation therapy, but they have a limited lifespan and may eventually require replacement.

3. Surgical Techniques:

Valve replacement surgery can be performed using two main approaches:

❖ **Open-Heart Surgery:** This involves making an incision in the chest, temporarily stopping the heart, and placing the patient on a heart-lung machine. The damaged valve is removed, and the new valve prosthesis is sewn into place.

❖ **Minimally Invasive Surgery:** In certain cases, valve replacement can be performed using minimally invasive techniques, which involve smaller incisions and specialized instruments. Minimally invasive approaches often result in reduced scarring, faster recovery, and shorter hospital stays.

4. Patient Selection:

The decision for valve replacement versus repair depends on several factors, including the type and severity of valve disease, overall health, age, lifestyle, and the expertise of the surgical team. In some cases, valve replacement may be the most appropriate treatment option.

5. Postoperative Care:

Following valve replacement surgery, patients require close monitoring and postoperative care. This includes medication management, regular follow-up visits, and adherence to lifestyle modifications.

Patients with mechanical valves need ongoing anticoagulation therapy, and all patients should be vigilant for any signs of complications or changes in symptoms.

Transcatheter Valve Interventions

Transcatheter valve interventions, also known as transcatheter valve therapies, are minimally invasive procedures used to treat certain types of valvular heart disease. These procedures involve the placement of a new valve within the diseased valve using a catheter, without the need for open-heart surgery. Here is a short and detailed overview of transcatheter valve interventions:

1. Purpose:

Transcatheter valve interventions are performed to address specific valve abnormalities, such as aortic stenosis or mitral regurgitation. These procedures aim to improve valve function, alleviate symptoms, and enhance overall heart function.

2. Types of Transcatheter Valve Interventions:

- *Transcatheter Aortic Valve Replacement (TAVR):*
  TAVR is used to treat severe aortic stenosis, where the aortic valve becomes narrowed.
  During the procedure, a new valve is delivered to the site of the diseased aortic valve through a catheter, usually inserted via the groin or chest. The new valve is expanded, pushing aside the old valve, and assumes its function.

- *Transcatheter Mitral Valve Repair (TMVR):*
  TMVR is performed to address mitral regurgitation, where the mitral valve fails to close properly, causing blood leakage.

This procedure uses specialized devices delivered through a catheter to repair the valve, improving its function and reducing regurgitation.

3. Procedure:

Transcatheter valve interventions are typically performed under local anesthesia or light sedation. The new valve or repair device is inserted into a catheter, which is guided through the blood vessels to the site of the diseased valve. The new valve is then positioned within the existing valve, either by expanding a collapsible valve or deploying a repair device. Once in place, the new valve or device assumes its function, improving valve function and blood flow.

4. Benefits:

Transcatheter valve interventions offer several advantages over traditional open-heart surgery, including:

- ❖ **Minimally Invasive:** These procedures are less invasive than open-heart surgery, resulting in smaller incisions, reduced trauma, and quicker recovery times.

❖ **Suitable for High-Risk Patients:** Transcatheter valve interventions are often suitable for patients who may not be candidates for open-heart surgery due to advanced age, multiple comorbidities, or frailty.

❖ **Shorter Hospital Stays:** Compared to open-heart surgery, transcatheter valve interventions typically require shorter hospital stays, allowing for faster recovery and return to normal activities.

5. Patient Selection:

Not all patients with valvular heart disease are candidates for transcatheter valve interventions. Patient selection depends on factors such as the type and severity of valve disease, anatomical considerations, overall health, and the expertise of the healthcare team. The decision for transcatheter valve intervention versus other treatment options is made on an individual basis.

Lifestyle Changes for Valvular Heart Disease

In addition to medical treatments, lifestyle changes are essential for managing valvular heart disease and improving overall heart health. These changes can help reduce symptoms, slow down the progression of the disease, and improve quality of life.

These lifestyle modifications for individuals with valvular heart disease include:

1. Healthy Diet:

Adopting a heart-healthy diet is crucial. Prioritize fruits, vegetables, whole grains, lean proteins, and low-fat dairy. Limit sodium (salt) intake to reduce fluid retention and blood pressure. Control portion sizes and avoid or limit saturated and trans fats, cholesterol, processed foods, and sugary beverages.

2. Regular Exercise:

Exercise regularly as advised by your doctor. Exercise helps strengthen the heart, improve cardiovascular fitness, control weight, and enhance overall well-being.

Discuss with your healthcare provider to determine the appropriate level and type of exercise for your condition.

3. Smoking Cessation:

Quit smoking and avoid secondhand smoke. Smoking increases the risk of heart disease and worsens symptoms in individuals with valvular heart disease. Seek professional help and support to quit smoking if needed.

4. Weight Management:

Maintain a healthy weight by combining frequent exercise with a well-balanced diet. Excess weight puts extra strain on the heart and can worsen symptoms of valvular heart disease.

5. Stress Management:

Practice stress-reducing techniques such as deep breathing exercises, meditation, yoga, or engaging in activities that promote relaxation. Chronic stress can adversely affect heart health, so it's important to find healthy ways to manage stress.

6. Medication Adherence:

Follow your doctor's instructions and take your medications regularly. Adhering to the recommended medication regimen is crucial for managing symptoms, controlling blood pressure, preventing complications, and improving overall heart function.

7. Regular Follow-up:

Attend regular follow-up appointments with your healthcare provider. Regular monitoring and assessment of your condition are essential to track progress, adjust treatment plans if needed, and address any concerns or changes in symptoms.

8. Health Education:

Educate yourself about valvular heart disease, its management, and warning signs of complications. Learn to recognize and respond to symptoms promptly, and seek medical attention when necessary.

9. Support Network:

Build a support network of family, friends, or support groups who understand and can provide emotional support during your journey with valvular heart disease.

Sharing experiences and connecting with others facing similar challenges can be helpful.

Adopting these lifestyle changes can have a positive impact on your heart health and overall well-being. Don't forget to speak with your healthcare provider to create a customized plan that works for your unique situation and needs. Your healthcare team can provide guidance, monitor your progress, and help you achieve optimal heart health.

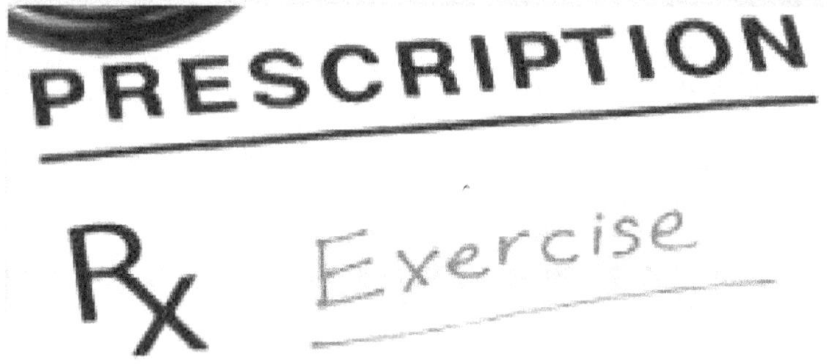

CHAPTER 6

Complications and Prognosis of Valvular Heart Disease

Valvular heart disease can lead to various complications that affect prognosis and overall health. Here is a short and detailed overview of the complications associated with valvular heart disease and the prognosis:

1. Complications:

- ❖ **Heart Failure:** Valvular heart disease can lead to heart failure, a condition in which the heart is unable to pump enough blood to meet the body's needs. It can result in symptoms such as shortness of breath, fatigue, fluid retention, and decreased exercise tolerance.

- ❖ **Arrhythmias:** Valve disease can disrupt the heart's normal electrical signals, leading to irregular heart rhythms (arrhythmias). These arrhythmias can cause palpitations, lightheadedness, fainting, and can potentially be life-threatening.

❖ **Infective Endocarditis:** Damaged heart valves are more prone to bacterial infections, leading to infective endocarditis. This condition can cause symptoms like fever, fatigue, joint pain, and can potentially damage the valves further.

❖ **Stroke and Blood Clots:** Certain types of valvular heart disease, such as mitral stenosis or atrial fibrillation, increase the risk of blood clot formation. If a clot dislodges and travels to the brain, it can cause a stroke, resulting in neurological deficits.

❖ **Pulmonary Hypertension:** Valvular heart disease, particularly affecting the mitral or tricuspid valves, can lead to increased pressure in the lungs (pulmonary hypertension). This can cause symptoms like shortness of breath, fatigue, and eventually right-sided heart failure.

❖ **Cardiac Arrest or Sudden Death:** In severe cases of valvular heart disease, particularly when left untreated or poorly managed, there is a risk of sudden cardiac arrest or sudden cardiac death.

This occurs when the heart suddenly stops functioning effectively, leading to a loss of consciousness and absence of a pulse.

Other Complications:

- ❖ Valvular heart disease can also contribute to other complications, such as heart valve rupture, heart valve thrombosis (clot formation on the valve), embolism (clot or debris dislodgement), heart valve calcification, or progressive deterioration of heart function.

2. Prognosis:

- ❖ The prognosis for valvular heart disease varies depending on several factors, including the specific type and severity of valve disease, the presence of symptoms, the response to treatment, and the overall health of the individual.
- ❖ With appropriate medical management and timely interventions, many individuals with valvular heart

disease can have a good prognosis and a relatively normal life expectancy.

❖ Early detection and treatment of valve disease are crucial in preventing complications and improving outcomes. Regular follow-up with a healthcare provider specializing in heart valve conditions is essential for monitoring the disease progression, optimizing treatment, and managing potential complications.

❖ The prognosis may be influenced by factors such as the underlying cause of valve disease, the ability to repair versus replace a valve, the choice of valve prosthesis if replacement is necessary, the individual's response to treatment, and the presence of other comorbidities.

❖ The prognosis can be improved with lifestyle modifications, adherence to prescribed medications, regular monitoring, and appropriate follow-up care.

It is important for individuals with valvular heart disease to work closely with their healthcare providers, follow the recommended treatment plan, and make necessary lifestyle changes. By managing the disease effectively, addressing complications promptly, and optimizing overall heart health, the prognosis for individuals with valvular heart disease can be significantly improved.

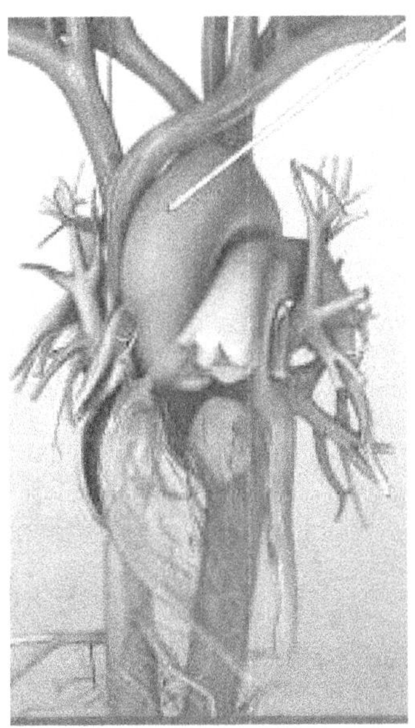

CHAPTER 7

Prevention and Management of Valvular Heart Disease

Prevention and effective management are essential for addressing valvular heart disease and reducing the risk of complications. Here is a short and detailed overview of the prevention and management strategies for valvular heart disease:

1. Prevention:

❖ **Maintain a Healthy Lifestyle:** Adopting a healthy lifestyle is crucial in preventing heart disease, including valvular heart disease. This includes following a balanced diet, engaging in regular physical activity, maintaining a healthy weight, avoiding smoking, and managing stress.

❖ **Regular Check-ups:** Regular medical check-ups allow healthcare providers to monitor your overall health, assess any risk factors for heart disease, and detect early signs of valve abnormalities.

Routine evaluations, including physical examinations and echocardiograms, can aid in early detection and intervention.

- ❖ Treat Underlying Conditions: Properly manage and treat conditions such as high blood pressure, high cholesterol, and diabetes, as these can contribute to the development and progression of valvular heart disease.

- ❖ Practice Good Oral Hygiene: Maintain good oral hygiene by regularly brushing and flossing your teeth and visiting your dentist for check-ups. Poor oral health and untreated dental infections can increase the risk of infective endocarditis, a serious complication of valvular heart disease.

2. Management:

- ❖ **Medications:** Depending on the specific type and severity of valvular heart disease, medications may be prescribed to manage symptoms, control blood pressure, prevent blood clots, or regulate heart rhythm. Adhering to the prescribed medication regimen is crucial for effective management.

❖ **Lifestyle Modifications:** Adopting a heart-healthy lifestyle is important for managing valvular heart disease. This includes following a nutritious diet, engaging in regular physical activity as recommended by your healthcare provider, maintaining a healthy weight, avoiding tobacco and excessive alcohol consumption, and managing stress.

❖ **Regular Follow-up:** Regular follow-up visits with your healthcare provider are essential for monitoring your condition, assessing treatment effectiveness, and making any necessary adjustments to the treatment plan.
Routine evaluations, such as echocardiograms and other diagnostic tests, help track the progression of the disease and detect any changes in valve function.

❖ **Surgical Interventions:** In some cases, surgical interventions may be necessary to repair or replace the diseased valve.

The decision for surgery depends on factors such as the severity of the valve disease, the presence of symptoms, and individual patient characteristics. It is important to discuss the benefits, risks, and expected outcomes of surgical interventions with your healthcare provider.

❖ **Emotional Support:** Living with valvular heart disease can be challenging. Seek emotional support from loved ones, join support groups, or consider counseling to cope with the emotional and psychological impact of the condition.

By following these preventive measures and effectively managing valvular heart disease, you can reduce the risk of complications, improve your overall heart health, and enhance your quality of life. Collaboration with healthcare providers and adherence to recommended treatments and lifestyle modifications are key to successful prevention and management of valvular heart disease.

Follow-up Care and Monitoring for Valvular Heart Disease

Regular follow-up care and monitoring are crucial for individuals with valvular heart disease to ensure optimal management and track the progression of the condition. Here is a short and detailed overview of follow-up care and monitoring for valvular heart disease:

1. Healthcare Provider Visits:

❖ **Regular Appointments:** Attend scheduled follow-up appointments with your healthcare provider who specializes in valvular heart disease. These visits allow for comprehensive evaluations, discussions about your symptoms, and adjustments to your treatment plan, if necessary.

❖ **Physical Examinations:** During each visit, your healthcare provider will conduct a physical examination to assess your heart sounds, check for any signs of fluid retention, and monitor your general health status.

❖ **Symptom Assessment:** Communicate any changes in your symptoms or the development of new symptoms to your healthcare provider. This information helps them assess the effectiveness of your treatment and determine if any adjustments are needed.

2. Diagnostic Testing:

❖ **Echocardiogram:** This non-invasive test uses sound waves to create images of your heart. It provides valuable information about the structure and function of your heart valves, helps evaluate any changes in valve function, and guides treatment decisions.

❖ **Electrocardiogram (ECG):** This test records the electrical activity of your heart. It helps detect any abnormal heart rhythms (arrhythmias) and assesses the overall electrical functioning of your heart.

❖ **Cardiac MRI or CT scan:** These imaging tests may be recommended to obtain more detailed images of your heart and assess the condition of your heart valves. They can provide valuable information about the size, shape, and function of your heart.

❖ **Stress Testing:** In some cases, stress testing may be performed to evaluate the heart's response to exercise or medication-induced stress. This test helps assess the functional capacity of your heart and determines if any exercise restrictions are necessary.

3. Medication Management:

❖ **Adherence to Medications:** Take prescribed medications as directed by your healthcare provider. Adhering to the recommended medication regimen is crucial for managing symptoms, controlling blood pressure, preventing complications, and improving overall heart function.

❖ **Medication Adjustments:** Your healthcare provider may periodically review your medications and adjust the dosages or types of medications based on your response to treatment, changes in your condition, or the development of any side effects.

4. Lifestyle Modifications:

❖ **Healthy Lifestyle:** Maintain a heart-healthy lifestyle by following a balanced diet, engaging in regular physical activity as recommended by your healthcare provider, managing stress, maintaining a healthy weight, and avoiding smoking and excessive alcohol consumption.

❖ **Regular Exercise:** Follow your healthcare provider's recommendations for exercise, which may include both aerobic exercises and strength training. Regular physical activity helps improve cardiovascular fitness, heart function, and overall well-being.

- ❖ **Weight Management:** Sustain a healthy weight by combining a balanced diet with frequent exercise. Achieving and maintaining a healthy weight reduces the strain on your heart and helps optimize your overall cardiovascular health.

- ❖ **Stress Management:** Adopt stress-reducing techniques such as deep breathing exercises, meditation, yoga, or engaging in activities that promote relaxation. Chronic stress can adversely affect heart health, so it's important to find healthy ways to manage stress.

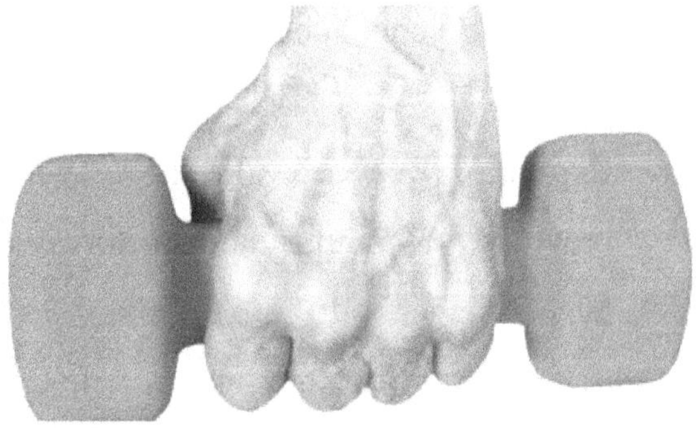

Living with Valvular Heart Disease

Being diagnosed with valvular heart disease requires adjustments and proactive management to lead a fulfilling life. Here is a short and detailed overview of living with valvular heart disease:

1. Education and Understanding:

Learn about your specific type of valvular heart disease, its causes, symptoms, and treatment options. Understanding your condition empowers you to actively participate in your care and make informed decisions.

2. Regular Medical Care:

Attend regular follow-up appointments with your healthcare provider who specializes in valvular heart disease. These visits help monitor your condition, assess treatment effectiveness, and make any necessary adjustments to your treatment plan.

3. Medication Management:

Take your doctor-prescribed medications.

Adhering to the recommended medication regimen is crucial for managing symptoms, controlling blood pressure, preventing complications, and improving overall heart function. Discuss all kind of side effects and concerns with your doctor.

4. Lifestyle Modifications:

Adopt a heart-healthy lifestyle by following a balanced diet, engaging in regular physical activity as recommended by your healthcare provider, maintaining a healthy weight, avoiding smoking, managing stress, and limiting alcohol consumption. These modifications help optimize heart health and overall well-being.

5. Emotional Support:

Living with valvular heart disease can be emotionally challenging. Seek support from loved ones, join support groups, or consider counseling to cope with the emotional and psychological impact of the condition. Openly discuss your feelings and concerns with your healthcare provider.

6. Self-Care:

Take care of your physical and emotional well-being. Get enough rest, manage stress through relaxation techniques, practice good oral hygiene, maintain a positive outlook, and engage in activities that bring joy and fulfillment.

7. Monitor Symptoms:

Pay attention to any changes in symptoms and report them to your healthcare provider. This helps in assessing the effectiveness of your treatment and making any necessary adjustments. Seek immediate medical attention for any sudden or severe symptoms.

8. Engage in Regular Physical Activity:

Follow your healthcare provider's recommendations for exercise, which may include aerobic exercises, strength training, or low-impact activities. Regular physical activity helps improve cardiovascular fitness, heart function, and overall well-being.

9. Communicate and Collaborate:

Keep lines of communication open and honest with your medical professional. Share your concerns, ask questions, and actively participate in decisions regarding your treatment plan. Engage in shared decision-making to ensure the best possible care.

10. Stay Positive and Seek Enjoyment:

Focus on the positive aspects of life and find joy in everyday activities. Engage in hobbies, spend time with loved ones, and pursue activities that bring you happiness and fulfillment. Maintaining a positive mindset can contribute to your overall well-being.

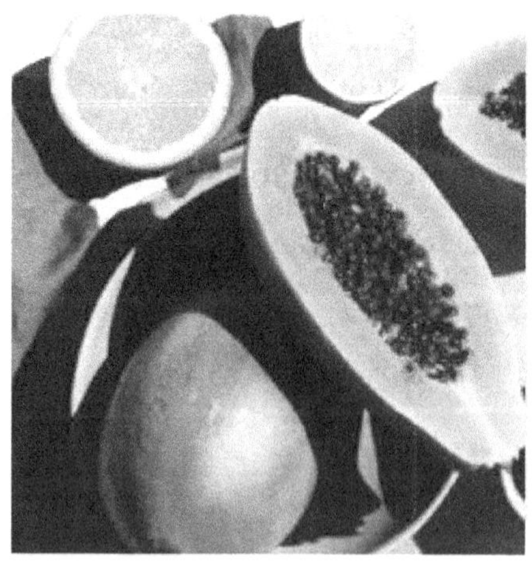

CONCLUSION

In conclusion, valvular heart disease refers to the dysfunction or damage of the heart valves, impairing the normal flow of blood within the heart. It can affect any of the four heart valves: the aortic valve, mitral valve, tricuspid valve, and pulmonary valve. Valvular heart disease can have various causes, including congenital defects, degenerative changes, infections, or rheumatic fever. It presents with a range of symptoms, such as shortness of breath, fatigue, chest pain, and swelling of the extremities.

Early diagnosis and appropriate management are crucial for individuals with valvular heart disease. Treatment options include medication management, lifestyle modifications, valve repair, or valve replacement. Regular follow-up care, monitoring, and adherence to treatment plans are essential to track disease progression, manage symptoms, and prevent complications. Engaging in a heart-healthy lifestyle can significantly improve outcomes.

Living with valvular heart disease requires self-care, emotional support, and collaboration with healthcare providers. By actively participating in one's care, staying informed, and seeking support, individuals with valvular heart disease can lead fulfilling lives while effectively managing their condition. It is important to work closely with healthcare professionals, attend regular check-ups, and communicate any changes in symptoms to ensure optimal management and long-term well-being.

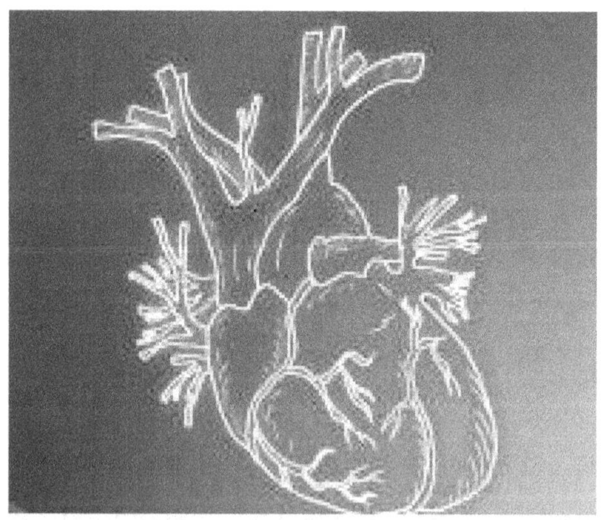